Conquer Colitis Now!

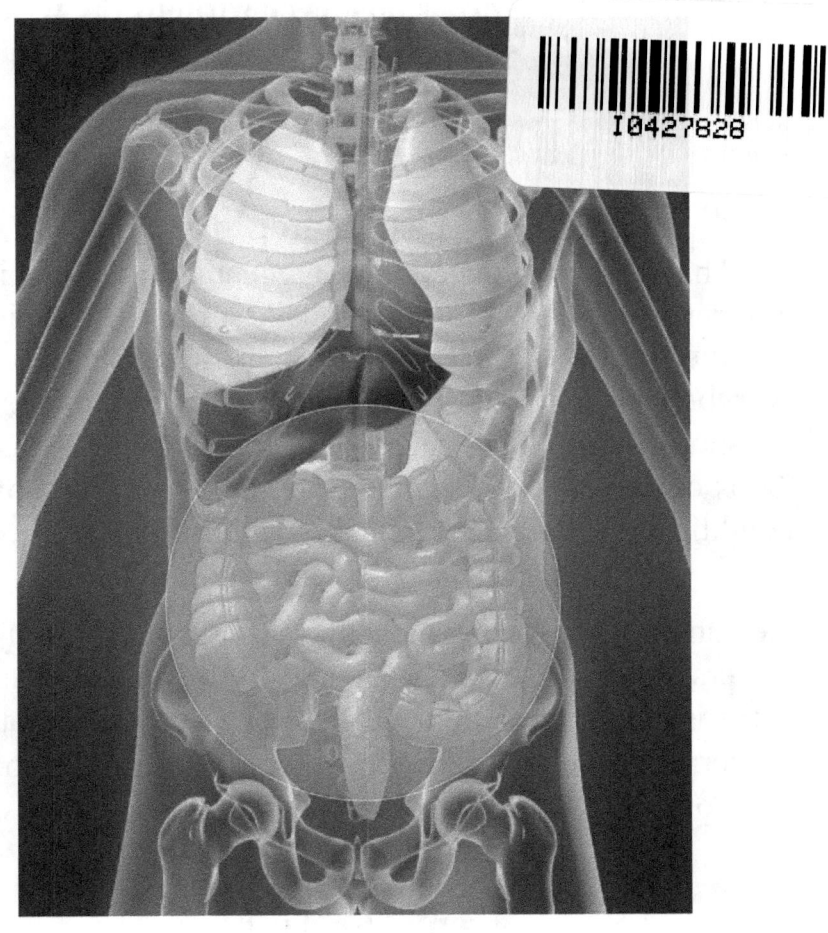

How To Treat Colitis & Live Pain Free For Life

Disclaimer

This book is intended to be a general guide, to raise awareness, and to help people make informed decisions in the context of their own personal circumstance. As everybody's circumstances are different, so are the remedies you should seek. While many of the recommendations in this book can be applied by almost anybody regardless of their conditions they are not intended to and should not be relied upon to replace personal medical advice.

The author accepts no responsibility for any loss or injury, be it personal or financial, as a result for the use or misuse of the information in this book. If you have any doubts or concerns after reading this book, please speak to a doctor or other qualified person before taking any actions.

From The Author

Thank you for taking the time to read this book. As an author, I understand the importance of creating books which my readers will find both enjoyable and informative. If you have the time and feel generous, please don't hesitate to leave an honest review of this book.........Dr Brad Turner.

Contents

Introduction

Chapter 1
Choosing The Right Food Plan

Chapter 2
Food You Should Avoid

Chapter 3
Food Supplements, Vitamins and Natural Remedies
For Colitis

Chapter 4
How To Avoid Emotional Stress

Chapter 5
Regular Exercise

Chapter 6
Additional Ways You Can Treat Colitis

Conclusion

Introduction

Over the last century, we observe a huge growth in the number of people suffering from all types of colitis, main form being the inflammatory bowel diseases (IBD). This growth is typical for developed and industrialized societies of Europe, Northern America and Australia. From estimated 28 patients per 100.000 people in early seventies, we are now dealing with approximately 199 patients per 100.000 people suffering from all types of colitis each year. Although the descriptions of bowel diseases resembling cases of Crohn's disease are present in the medical literature from sixteenth century, they have not become a subject of analysis until past few decades. Growing incidence and difficulties with proper diagnosing and treating of inflammatory bowel diseases were the reasons, why many studies were made over the last few decades in order to determine the causes and risk factors for these diseases. After many years of hard work, we are still not much closer to getting answers to our questions about IBD. The most popular theory, which is trying to explain why people suffer from IBD's is hygiene hypothesis. Over the last few decades, we developed many new ways to improve our food storage conditions and to preserve our food, making it eatable for a longer period of time. That, and also decreased level of consumed food contamination, are the reasons, why the overall frequency of enteric infections has decreased. Without having something to fight with (in that case, that would be all the pathogens causing enteric infections), our immune system responsible for taking care of our digestive system starts to overreact - when a pathogen, that in a healthy person would cause only a little inflammatory response that would limit itself and not cause any trouble, shows up in digestive system of susceptible host, it triggers an overwhelming immune response, that leads to chronic inflammations of most of digestive tract. Of course, now we should ask who these susceptible hosts are. Many studies indicate, that there are genes, which may be responsible for susceptibility to those kinds of overwhelming inflammatory responses.

This is just one of many theories trying to explain the complex nature of Inflammatory Bowel Diseases. If we were to tell the actual state of our knowledge about IBD's, we would say that these diseases are idiopathic, which means that the processes responsible for them are not yet discovered. Right now the scientists believe that Inflammatory Bowel Diseases originate from a combination of dysfunction of intestinal epithelium, immune mucosal tissues overreaction and some defects in host interaction with intestinal micro biota. All those factors combined may produce a disease in a susceptible host.

The image of IBD's is not yet optimistic. But if we remember the 90's, we may see that cardiovascular diseases were a similar problem. Origins were not well known, we were not that good at treating them, but after few years we became capable of managing them.

One of the factors, that was so important and of great significance in our fight with cardiovascular diseases was patient's self-awareness and their ability to control risk factors responsible for the rapid onset of cardiovascular diseases on their own at their homes. It quickly revealed, that if properly educated, people can easily modify their lifestyle and become „immune" to cardiovascular diseases - by choosing a right diet or starting to exercise.

We believe, that self awareness, proper diet and managing of all yet known risk factors of IBD's are the key to deal with this epidemic. This is why this book is written - to show patients what can be done by themselves, at their homes, in order to prevent the disease, to ease its natural course, or not allow it to spread. First part of this book will describe all the types of Inflammatory Bowel Diseases, its pathogenesis and natural course if untreated. Second part will be the demonstration of all dietary possibilities, physical exercises and other supplements helpful in dealing with IBD's. We believe that it will be both educating and easy to understand and as a result will help patients in managing their disease.

About Inflammatory Bowel Diseases

Inflammatory Bowel Diseases comprises two main diseases: Crohn's disease and Ulcerative Colitis. Many scholars argue about what are the factors, which led to the onset of the disease. Also it is unsure, if Crohn's disease and Ulcerative Colitis are two different diseases, with different pathogenesis, course and outcome, or if they are two different results of the same disease. There are still many questions unanswered about Inflammatory Bowel Diseases. What they both have in common, is that they are a result of misregulation between three factors: intestinal microbiota, intestinal epithelium and the immune system. They differ in many ways as well: the regions of colon they attack, layers of intestine wall that is in the state of inflammation, natural course and complications.

Crohn's disease typically begins at the age of 20. Its clinical manifestations are extremely variable, and include: intermittent attacks of mild diarrheal, fever and abdominal pain. In about 20% of the patients, it mimics acute appendicitis: right lower quadrant pain, fever and bloody diarrheal. Active period of the disease are typically interrupted by asymptomatic periods. Emotional stress, dietary mistakes or cigarette smoking are associated with the disease re-activation. It can attack all parts of intestines such as: small intestine or colon. The distribution of lesions is skippy, which means that only parts of the intestines are affected. The inflammatory process covers all the depth of the intestinal wall.

Ulcerative colitis on the other hand, is limited only to the colon and rectum. Its distribution is diffuse, and the inflammatory process is limited only to mucosal layer of the intestinal wall. Its typical clinical features are attacks of blood, diarrhea, lower abdominal pain and cramps, which are temporarily relieved by defecation. What is interesting, is that smoking cessation is the reason for disease's onset in some patients, and smoking may partially relieve the symptoms of the disease. Emotional stress and dietary mistakes are the factors that lead to disease's re-activation. Both of these can be managed by dietary restrictions, physical activity, and stress management.

Chapter 1

Choosing The Right Food Plan

First, what comes to mind, when managing diseases of gastrointestinal tract is choosing a proper diet. Inflammatory Bowel Disease is no different.

One of the factors, believed to trigger the initial overwhelming immune reaction in our gastrointestinal tract is the consumption of highly processed and preserved food. Amazing as it may seem, our dietary habits have changed incredibly over the last two thousand years. Our bodies possess unimaginable possibilities for adapting to the changes of the environment we live in. If we say, that over a century, three generations pass, and each of these passes is a possibility to our set of genes to rebuild, then our genome had only sixty possibilities to adapt to changes over the last two thousand years. Even for such an amazing machine,, sixty genetic shifts are not enough to adapt to our rapidly changing dietary habits. As a result, we are not fully genetically adapted to the food we are consuming.

The basis of our daily menu is composed of highly processed food, rich in preservatives. The amount of dietary fiber consumed is decreasing. Dietary fiber is responsible for proper bowel movement, and thus is an exceptionally important factor in preventing bowel disease. On the other hand, dietary fiber stimulates the mucosal layer in our intestines to produce mucus and other layers to produce enzymes needed to digest etc. In a healthy man, this plays an extremely important role in the correct functioning of our digestive system. However, what is good for a healthy person, is not for a patient already suffering from IBD, where a production of mucus and enzymes by a weakened bowel wall further impairs its function and exacerbates the course of the disease. High intake of preservatives particles results in "confusion" of our immune system, especially its part localized in digestive system. Low consumption of dietary fiber results in the impairment of bowel movements and the weakening of the intestinal wall. This weakening is an important factor, contributing to the development of Inflammatory Bowel Disease. The immune system is starting to have problems with differentiating between microbial pathogens, chemical particles present in preservatives and the body's own tissues. After some time, this misregulation may result in our immune system not being able to contain itself, and when a pathogen, that normally would not cause any harm to our digestive tract, enters the colon, an overwhelming inflammatory reaction occurs, and results in chronic inflammatory reaction, which typically results in Inflammatory Bowel Disease.

Now we see why a proper diet is such an important factor in keeping us healthy. Our genes are programmed to deal with food not processed, as most of us consume. As we remember, we are genetically prepared to consume foods that were typical around two thousand years ago. The food back then was far more contaminated, which resulted in a high incidence of bacterial colonitis, but had this advantage, that the immune system localized in our intestines had something to fight with all the time. Now our food is clean and processed, which is a fantastic thing, because we have eliminated many deadly infectious diseases; but at a price of misregulations in our digestive tracts' immune system. Patients suffering from colonitis may be able to control their symptoms by applying to few dietary rules. As we can see from above, intake of preservatives and processed food is one of the reasons Inflammatory Bowel Disease occurs in the first place. Some dietary changes may ease the course of the disease. Here are dietary suggestions helpful in dealing with Inflammatory Bowel Disease:

1. It is highly advisable to decrease the consumption of raw fruits and vegetables; the suggested amount of eating fruits and vegetables is five times a day, but they should be boiled, peeled etc. One should eliminate fruits containing stones, such as apples, pears, plums etc.;

2. One should limit the amount of red meat consumed, as it is not as easily digested as white meat, like chicken or turkey; overall consumption of protein should increase;

3. Decrease the amount of dietary fiber in our daily menu; especially rich sources of fiber: full grain wheat, dark bread, bananas, pineapples, beans, soy, bran, raspberries; it may seem illogical, because lack of dietary fiber is thought to be one of the reasons why the disease occurs in first place, but on second thought it makes a lot of sense; big amounts of fiber result in bigger production of feces; defecation in patients suffering from IBD's is very painful and problematic, also bigger feces production may further impair bowel wall function, which is already heavily impaired;

4. It is highly advisable to limit the amount of preserved food consumed;

5. One should try to decrease the amount of fat in daily diet;
6. Alcohol should be eliminated;

7. One should try to limit the amount of spices used in cooking;

8. It is better to avoid frying food or roasting it;

Applying these rules in your everyday routine will be helpful in relieving symptoms of Inflammatory Bowel Disease. Of course, what is important, is that some of the products, which are healthy and should be eaten during the course of the disease, may aggravate the symptoms in some patients; the most important thing is to observe the body and avoid foods that worsen the symptoms. What is even more important, is the decrease in consumption of dietary fiber, as it may worsen the course of the disease, as mentioned before. Diet of a patient suffering from an IBD should contain decreased quantity of fiber, should be around 2000-3000 kcal per day, contain high amount of protein (80-120 g per day), and also decreased amount of fat (maximum at a level 50-70g per day). Patients should eat small portions of food 5-6 times a day instead of eating huge meals 3 times a day. During the onset or the exacerbation of the disease, which typically manifests as heavy diarrhea, it is preferable to consume liquid forms of food, such as carrot pure, blackberry jelly, and to drink a high amount of water or isotonic drinks, to compensate for everything lost during diarrhea. Liquid food is digested quickly and does not irritate the bowels. After 3-4 days, when sudden symptoms start to disappear, one can begin with a normal diet, mentioned above.

If we were to summarise the dietary rules, which are to be obeyed in the course of Inflammatory Bowel Disease, we can say that it should be a diet of a healthy man. Non-processed food, low intake of fats is the thing everyone should do when it comes to the way they eat. These rules are especially important when it comes to the digestive tract diseases, when its function is impaired. Patients should also avoid all of the food which aggravates the course of the disease. Typical food that is suggested in the course of IBD is listed below:

- white bread;
- skimmed milk, skimmed cheese;
- soft-boiled eggs;
- chicken, turkey;
- fishes with low fat amount;
- olive oil;
- carrot, spinach, lettuce, tomato;
- tea;
- jellies, waffles, honey;

As mentioned before, it is extremely important to observe how our body reacts to different foods and eliminate everything that makes us feel worse.

Chapter 2

Food You Should Avoid

If we look at dietary suggestions, it becomes clear, what type of food should be avoided by patients suffering from Inflammatory Bowel Disease. Food that is rich in dietary fiber, such as whole grain bread, bran, many fruits and vegetables, for example bananas, pineapples, beans soy, is not recommended in the course of Inflammatory Bowel Disease, especially during the period of exacerbation of the disease, as it may worsen the symptoms and make the process of getting better difficult.

Anything, that irritates our digestive system, should be avoided at any cost, as it may provoke a sudden onset of heavy symptoms. Hot spices, alcohol are the things that are well known of its role in provoking disease exacerbations. Anything that is difficult to digest also should be avoided. Mushrooms, raw fruits and vegetables need some time to be digested, and the longer the food stays in our digestive tract, the bigger the chances of irritating the intestinal wall are, and the risk of exacerbation of the course of the disease is getting bigger.

Typically, the IBDs start and relapse as heavy diarrhea. It is critical during that period to avoid any types of solid foods, as their contact with the intestinal wall during the process of digestion irritates it.

Below is a list of food products that should be avoided by the patients suffering from Inflammatory Bowel Disease:
- whole grain wheat and bread;
- milk, cream, cheese;
- fried eggs;
- pork, duck, goose, bacon;

- fishes containing a lot of fat;
- canned fish;
- crisps and chips;
- pepper, mustard, chilli;
- chocolate, cakes;
- coffee and alcohol;

It is very important to obey the rules and suggestions mentioned above, as the consumption of inappropriate food may worsen the course of the disease and make the process of getting better very difficult.

Chapter 3

Food Supplements, Vitamins and Natural Remedies For Colitis

Inflammatory Bowel Diseases lasts for many years. During the course of the diseases, we observe periods of relapse and exacerbations. The intestinal wall is under a lot of pressure from our immune system, from the food we consume, from the stress we live in. All these factors weaken the intestinal wall, which in turn, becomes less and less capable of digesting and absorbing the food we consume. But we consume not only the food; vitamins, microelements and ions are also present in our diet, and they play an extremely important role in the proper functioning of our body. With our intestine weakened, it is almost impossible to provide our organism with the amount of vitamins and microelements it needs. Normally, our everyday diet brings enough vitamins and microelements to satisfy our body's needs, but when it comes to Inflammatory Bowel Disease, when our intestines are weak and are not able to absorb food properly, the amount of vitamins absorbed is insufficient. That is why it is so important to supplement our body in the proper way.

The most important microelement necessary for the proper production and function of our erythrocytes, that is our blood's red cells, responsible for supplying our tissues with the oxygen they need, is iron.

In the course of Inflammatory Bowel Disease, after few years and cycles of exacerbations and relapses, our intestines finally end up in a state of malabsorption, that is a state when the process of absorption is impaired, and the body cannot be provided with the microelements it needs.

One of the first victims of this process is iron. When the

levels of iron in our body decrease, the first thing that is affected is the erythrocyte system. The number of red blood cells decrease, which manifests in chronic fatigue, easy bruising, not being able to get a good night sleep, shortness of breath, lower exertion tolerance, finally syncope's and in the cases of severe iron deficiency, the need to be hospitalized. In order to not allow the body to get to the state of severe iron deficiency, patients need to supplement iron in their diet. What is important, is to take an iron pill together with vitamin C, as it enables more iron to be absorbed. The amount of iron that needs to be taken daily should be assessed by a medical doctor, after a precise verification of iron levels in the patient's body.

Other vitamins that need to be supplemented are vitamins from the B group, the vitamins C, D, E and K. Every patient should use some multivitamin supplements, which are comprised of many different vitamins in an easy to absorb form. These kinds of supplements contain every vitamin and microelement needed, and should be a basis for every patient to start with. Additional supplementing should be done by a doctor, after a verification of levels of vitamins and microelements.

During the exacerbation period of the disease, when heavy diarrhea is one of the most important symptom, and heavy loss of microelements is typical, it is extremely important to take care of sufficient watering of our body. The best are isotonic drinks, which are full of microelements such as sodium and potassium, which are lost during the diarrheal. Isotonic drinks that can be purchased in a normal shop are not recommended, because they are not designed for patients. It is best to buy the needed supplement in the pharmacy, where we can be sure to get something designed to help ill people.

Natural remedies and colitis

As always, when a disease occurs, many so-called specialists claim to have an ultimate cure for it, and usually want a lot of money for their services, but don't always guarantee the results wanted by the patient.

Inflammatory Bowel Disease is no different. The internet is full of miracle substances that can cure patients of everything. We must stay very careful and alert, because some of the methods described on the internet not only don't do us any good, but may cause serious harm to the patient and make the process of getting better extremely difficult.

We will not discuss every natural remedy for colitis and especially for Inflammatory Bowel Disease that can be found on-line, because for most of them there are no proofs that they possibly work.

Some medical investigations show on the other hand, that consumption of dairy products, which contain natural bacterial flora, is beneficial for the patients suffering from the Inflammatory Bowel Disease.

Natural bacterial flora, present in some of the dairy products, help bring balance to the microbiota already present in our intestines. As we remember from our previous discussion, misbalance in intestinal flora is thought to be one of the causes of the disease in first place, so looking to restore that balance is an important direction of therapy.

We need to remember though, not to rely totally on just one possible treatment. Consumption of dairy products with natural bacterial flora should always be a part of a diet, and such a diet should be consulted with a physician or nutritionist first. Any information that we find about possible remedies should be taken cautiously. Any type of remedy should not be implemented until careful consultation with a doctor.

Using unprescribed drugs or other remedies can bring harm to our health and further aggravate the course of the disease, making it hard to control. In some cases, the use of drugs or remedies from unknown sources may be the cause of many new dangerous complications, which may have deadly consequences.

Chapter 4

How To Avoid Emotional Stress

As mentioned before, one of the many factors responsible for aggravating symptoms of the disease is stress. It was an extremely important factor during the early phases of the development of the human race, as it enabled us to react quickly to dangerous situations we found ourselves in. Stress as a short acting agent is a positive thing, as it allows us to adapt to some of the quick changes in our surroundings. But, if we allow stress to act for a long period of time, it starts to have a negative impact on us. Not only affects it our minds, but also bodies. The effects of prolonged stress vary depending on the organ it affects. Chronic fatigue, depression, anhedony, are the most common effects the stress has on our minds.

When it comes to the way it affects our internal organs, the symptoms are far more variable. Stress activates the sympathetic nervous system, which prepares our body to either "run or fight". When it comes specifically to the way it affects our digestive system, here is what it does: it stops the bowel movement, inhibits secretion and absorption, and also inhibits all the digestive processes. In the immobilized bowel, blood flow is also impaired, which is a situation that enables thinning of the intestinal wall: a tissue without proper blood flow is incapable of growing properly. As a result of living in chronic stress, we are unable to digest the food we consume properly, what's more, the thinning of the intestinal wall is the factor that facilitates the development of Inflammatory Bowel Disease.

When we look at all of these, we can clearly see, that developing ways to deal with the stress that we have to live in everyday is an extremely important thing to do, in order to prevent the development of Inflammatory Bowel Disease and ease its progress.

What can each and every one of us do to reduce the stress? There are many ways to deal with stress.

Regular physical exercises are known of its relaxing effects on both mind and body. Positive impact regular exercises have on patients suffering from Inflammatory Bowel Disease will be discussed further on.

One of the methods which is very effective in fighting with negative stress effects is meditation. In western countries it is popular among people interested in eastern cultures, but still not very well known to the majority of society. Regular meditation has a positive impact on the way our brain works - it improves our concentration, allows us to be able to focus better on what is happening inside our thoughts thus making us "immune" to the external world and as a result, allow us to deal with stress more efficiently. There are many different methods of meditation, each focusing on different things. There are sound meditations, guided meditations, so-called "five senses meditation" - each is very good in managing stress, but requires some professional guidance and assistance especially for beginners. The easiest type of meditation which can be done at home without any external help is called relaxation meditation. The whole idea of this exercise is to relax, sit in a comfortable position, and try not to concentrate on any specific thought. It may sound easy, but in fact not concentrating on anything specific is a bit of a challenge. It usually requires some time to get to that point, but it is worth it. What is important is to start with short sessions, from 5 to 10 minutes a day, and do sessions on regular basis. Very quickly you will see positive results.

If we do not feel that meditation is something adequate for us, but feel like emotional stress is something overwhelming, we can try attending some psychotherapy sessions. These may be very helpful in learning how to manage stress, but need to be done by a certified and qualified psychotherapist. As we see, learning how to deal with stress in our life is not an easy thing to do. There are many ways that can be helpful, physical and mental exercises, and both are very important. Managing stress is an important factor in easing symptoms of many diseases, including Inflammatory Bowel Disease, so it is very important to find a way of dealing with it. Not only will it reduce negative symptoms of the disease, but will allow patients to recover faster and will improve the quality of their lives.

Chapter 5

Regular Exercise

There are many different articles, stating how important and beneficial to our health regular exercise is. It is almost impossible to stress that enough. We cannot say that we are healthy, if we are not exercising. Regular movement helps us prevent many dangerous diseases. It is one of the most important factors in preventing cardiovascular diseases. Inflammatory Bowel Disease is no different.

One of the ways, by which regular exercises works positively on our bodies, is that it improves the blood flow in the tissues. Blood carries the oxygen, the glucose, microelements - basically, everything that a tissue needs to grow and repair itself.

Without proper blood flow, the tissues become slowly ischemic. That state impairs their function and after a longer period of time, tissue becomes weakened and does not function properly. That is what is happening in our digestive system when we do not get enough movement. In susceptible patients, it is one of the reasons why Inflammatory Bowel Disease occurs in the first place.

When we start moving, blood flow helps the tissue renew and grow stronger. It is an important factor in Inflammatory Bowel Disease, where the intestinal wall is weakened and does not function properly, thus physical exercises accelerate the process of getting better in the patients suffering from IBD.

One of the main rules, the patient suffering from Inflammatory Bowel Disease should obey when it comes to physical exercises, is that the level of exertion should be adequate to one's possibilities. Patients, who already had three operations because of Crohn's disease, never had run for more than fifteen minutes, cannot start their physical exercises plan by running ten kilometres in less than an hour. Everything has to be natural and cannot further aggravate the symptoms of the disease.

A reasonable plan to start any kind of physical activity in patients suffering from chronic diseases is to gradually bring the levels of exertion up.

Patients should start their activity only after having consulted a physician. Recommended activities in the beginning are walking 15-20 minutes a day. For example, instead of taking a bus or a tram to work, leave 20 minutes early and walk. Instead of using elevator to take you to the second floor, use the stairs. These are really simple things, but are a great way to start.

If you feel like you can do more, try light jogging, or take a yoga class. These are great activities that act on your whole body, and improve your well-being. They strengthen all of your body's muscles, your heart, and pulmonary system and improve functioning of your digestive system. As before, do not start anything new on a high level of exertion. Gradually intensify your trainings. After two to three months, you will see that whole your body is stronger you can tolerate the exertion better, digest better, and generally feel better. Of course, when it comes to the acute phase of the disease, any type of physical activity is not recommended, as it may worsen the course of the disease and make the process of getting better even harder. Mild physical activity is necessary in preventing the disease and controlling its course during the phase of relapse. If you feel that the physical exercises are not doing any good, then do not continue to do them. As in every aspect of the disease - the diet, the supplements, the stress management, the most important thing with the physical exercise is common sense. Every activity we plan to take on, should first be consulted by a physician, because

23

unwillingly, we may worsen the course of our disease.

Chapter 6

Additional Ways You Can Treat Colitis

Signs and symptoms that should make you consult a physician

As with every chronic disease, Inflammatory Bowel Disease should be managed by a qualified physician, who will be able to help in case the attack of the disease strikes. It is extremely important to obey the dietary rules, exercise, manage stress, generally take care of one's self, but there are times, that prevention and good lifestyle will not be able to help us.

Crohn's disease and Ulcerative Colitis are mysterious diseases, which are known to attack the patient surprisingly. Some patients may have two mild attacks during their whole life, whereas there are some, whose relapse period lasts only as long as two weeks, and they spend most of their times in hospitals.

It is important not to hesitate to consult a physician when we observe that the disease is starting to have a dangerous course. Typically, attacks of both of these diseases take the form of strikes of bloody diarrhea, fever and abdominal pain. The truth is that every attack of the disease should be a warning sign, and no one should disregard it. It is a reason to be admitted to the hospital, where a number of additional tests need to be performed. Every amount of blood in the feces is dangerous, and the reasons why they happened should be investigated. Bleeding from the digestive tract is dangerous as it may be very difficult to stop, and sometimes the bleeding continues, even though the blood is no longer visible in the feces. It happens, when it is absorbed back in the digestive tract. Nevertheless, it is crucial to find the source of bleeding in order to stop it.

High fever is also dangerous, especially when it exceeds the temperature of 40 Celsius degrees. That temperature is not only deadly for our bodies proteins, but also that type of fever, associated especially with abdominal pain, may be a symptom of peritoneitis, which a state that is life threatening state and should be immediately surgically treated.

Abdominal pain, that lasts for days, and moves from the center of the abdomen to the right side, associated with mild temperature, that typically does not exceed 38 Celsius degree may be the symptom of appendicitis, which, if untreated may also lead to peritoneitis.

Interestingly, Inflammatory Bowel Disease: Crohn's Disease and Ulcerative Colitis, may produce symptoms not only from the digestive tract. Polyarthritis, which is the inflammatory state that can be observed in many different joints at a one time, sacroilitis, which is an inflammation of the joints in the lower back, producing pain, especially when bending over, uveitis, skin lesions and primary sclerosis cholangitis, are the most common extra-intestinal manifestations of both Crohn's disease and Ulcerative Colitis. Bearing in mind, that genetics has its impact on the disease, we should remember, if any of our relatives are suffering from Inflammatory Bowel Disease, and we suffer from one of the diseases listed above, we are at a high risk of developing Inflammatory Bowel Disease and should consult a physician.

As we can see, the symptoms of aggravation of the Inflammatory Bowel Disease cannot be left without investigation and further treatment. What is more, every attack should be consulted by a physician, as some change in the treatment plan may be needed. Additional difficulty connected to managing of Inflammatory Bowel Disease is that it does not always produce symptoms from the gastrointestinal tract. That is why it is so important to stay alert and observe the way our body reacts, so that we can react properly when difficult time comes. On the other hand, we cannot forget how important it is to stick to the diet and try to avoid all the factors that may ease the aggravation of the disease. If we stick to all these rules, management of Inflammatory Bowel Disease will be a much easier job.

Conclusion

As we can see, not everything is known about the colonitis, especially about Inflammatory Bowel Disease. They are complex diseases, where many factors play important roles. Misregulations of many systems are a significant part of Inflammatory Bowel Disease pathogenesis. Genetics seem to play a very important role in how the disease will affect, making the search of susceptibility genes a future of possible cures for the disease.

Right now, there are many things that a patient can do on their own, in order to control the disease and make its course more bearable. Proper diet seems to be the key to avoiding attacks of the disease. When combined with physical exercise and stress management, it looks like most of the known trigger factors for attacks of the disease are eliminated. It is very important to observe how the body reacts to different agents, and avoid everything that makes the course of the disease more difficult.

Right now, we cannot say that one can be cured from Inflammatory Bowel Disease. They may have a remission lasting for many years, but we should still remember that the disease can strike at any time. That is why it is so important not to lose contact with your physician, since they will be able to help. Keeping a healthy balance between self-awareness, observing your own body, sticking to the chosen diet, avoiding all the negative factors and regular medical assistance seems to be the right way to deal with all outcomes of the disease.

Hopefully, the future will unveil answers we still keep asking about Inflammatory Bowel Diseases, as it has previously done with many deadly diseases, which now can be treated with a single pill.

Other Books By Dr Brad Turner

Headache Cures Made Easy

Headaches are extremely common, especially in today's society where everyone is stressed, exhausted and forever taking on too much work. However, the big problem arises when we stop viewing headaches as something serious. Whether large or small, headaches can often be a symptom of a more severe underlying problem and ignoring them is the worst thing we can do. Whether you regularly experience primary or secondary headaches, you can use this guide to 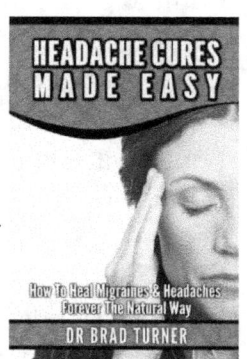 learn about the causes of headaches, the symptoms that can arise and how to tackle them if they are a common occurrence in your life. It also offers you details of natural cures, giving you useful tips and ideas to help stop that headache in its tracks, as well as information on how to prevent getting headaches and migraines in the future.

Lose Belly Fat Without Exercise

Dr Brad Turner's *Lose Belly Fat Without Exercise* is an easy to follow guide which gives you the important information you need to give you a jump start to a vibrant, radiant and sexy new you!

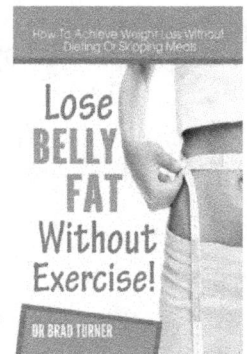

If you are tired of counting calories, fat grams and points and or have lost your motivation with crash course Exercise programs and are tired of diets that just do not work, then this book is for you.

The Type 2 Diabetes Cure

TYPE 2 DIABETES CURE just blew the myths out of the water concerning diabetes. It's the ultimate guide to diabetes, no matter the type. By defining all three types of diabetes, the author helps readers understand just how easy it is to overcome type 2 diabetes. From the sampling of mouth-watering recipes to eating plans, to exercise recommendations—TYPE 2 DIABETES CURE tells the truth--type 2 diabetes can be cured as well as prevented. And, that, my friends, is the most wonderful message in the book! Get your copy today and start your journey to incredible health.

Quit Smoking Naturally

On every literary corner, there's an expert on how to quit smoking. But very few of their theories stick. Every day the weary smoker is inspired to quit, only to have his/her hopes dashed yet again. *Quit Smoking Naturally* is the book that may set everyone free! The genius of this book is the straightforward approach and authentic voice that provides the facts, dispels the fallacies and motivates the smoker to do what they've never done before—succeed at quitting!

Natural Antibiotics And Antiviral For Beginners

Herbal Antibiotics and Antiviral for Beginners gives a very clear description of the types and uses of medicinal herbs all over the country. This book simply reminds us about how useful the herbs were during the times of our forefathers. As the name suggests, this book is a guide on herbal antibiotics and antiviral for the beginners. This book is a record of the various medical herbs and their properties. It also entails the preparations of the medicines from these herbs. Herbal medicines have the capacity of curing infections and diseases in the most convenient way. Not only that, but they are also almost completely harmless and have no side-effects whatsoever. The need for such medicines has become very intense since our bodies have developed a capacity to get used to the synthetic medicines.

The Adrenal Fatigue Cure

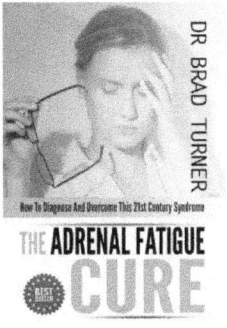

The average person knows little about adrenal fatigue let alone where the adrenal glands are located on the body. Situated above the kidneys, these glands, if not working properly, can hinder the function of all the other organs in the body. ADRENAL FATIGUE is an exemplary guide to the adrenal glands—from the symptoms of malfunctioning glands, to adrenal fatigue, even providing an easy to follow diet of delicious foods and beverages that will lead to healthy adrenal glands. ADRENAL FATIGUE should be in every home library. Get your copy today and start the journey to incredible health!

www.ingramcontent.com/pod-product-compliance
Lightning Source LLC
Chambersburg PA
CBHW070246290526
45789CB00004B/1793